OVERCOM
MULTIPLE SCLEROSIS

The Comprehensive Guide to Managing MS and living Your best Life

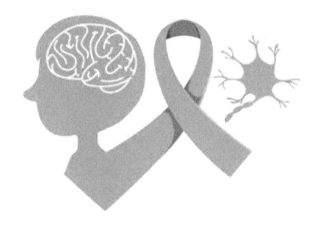

Vivian Ross

This book is a labor of love and the result of countless hours of research and dedication. It is the author's hope that the information contained within these pages will inspire and enlighten readers, and contribute to a better understanding of Multiple Sclerosis.

TABLE OF CONTENTS

Defeating Multiple Sclerosis isn't just about healing the body, it's about empowering the mind and spirit too...

Vivian Ross

INTRODUCTION

Sophie had always been an incredibly active person. She loved nothing more than going for long walks in the countryside, cycling, and even running the occasional marathon. So when she started to feel more and more tired as she entered her mid-thirties, she knew something was wrong.

At first, Sophie tried to ignore her symptoms. She told herself that she was just getting older, and that everyone got tired sometimes. But as the months went by, her balance became increasingly shaky, and she started to experience tingling sensations in her arms and legs.

It wasn't until Sophie went to see her doctor that she received the devastating news that she had multiple sclerosis. She was completely blindsided by the diagnosis, and she felt like her whole world had come crashing down around her.

Sophie knew that multiple sclerosis could be an incredibly debilitating disease, and she feared that it would rob her of everything she loved. She started to feel increasingly isolated and alone, as she struggled to come to terms with what was happening to her body. It was a dark time for her, and she felt as though there was no hope.

But then, one day, while she was browsing in her local library, she stumbled across a book that would change her life. The book, Overcoming Multiple Sclerosis was written by someone who had also been diagnosed with multiple sclerosis, but who had managed to live a full and active life despite their condition.

Sophie was initially hesitant to read the it, fearing that it would be yet another unhelpful self-help book. But as she started to flip through the pages, she began to realize that this was different.

It was incredibly detailed, and it was filled with practical advice for managing the symptoms of multiple sclerosis. It emphasized the importance of taking a holistic approach, and it focused on lifestyle changes that could make a real difference.

Sophie devoured the book, reading it from cover to cover in just a few days. She was amazed by the wealth of information it contained, and by how practical and easy-to-follow the advice was. She felt like she finally had a roadmap for how to live her life with multiple sclerosis, rather than just surviving from one day to the next.

As she began to put the advice into practice, Sophie started to notice a real difference in how she felt. She was less tired, her balance was improving, and she felt more in control of her condition. She was even able to start going for short walks again, something she had thought would never be possible.

Sophie's newfound sense of hope and control was incredibly empowering, and she soon became an evangelist for the book she had found. She started recommending it to anyone who would listen, both online and in person. She even set up a local support group for people living with multiple sclerosis, where she shared her story and encouraged others to take control of their condition.

Through it all, Sophie remained incredibly grateful for the book that had changed her life. She knew that multiple sclerosis was still a serious condition, and that there would be challenges ahead. But thanks to the approach she had discovered, she felt like she had the tools to face those challenges head-on, and to live her life to the fullest.

Looking back, Sophie knew that discovering the book had been a turning point in her life. It had given her hope, purpose, and a sense of community that she had never known before. And she was grateful every day for the simple but powerful message of the book: that even in the face of adversity, there is always hope, and always a way forward.

In the months that followed, Sophie continued to make positive changes to her lifestyle, all based on the advice she had found in the book. She started eating a healthier diet, focused on getting plenty of exercise, and even began practicing mindfulness and meditation.

Multiple Sclerosis (MS) is a chronic autoimmune disease that affects the central nervous system, causing a wide range of symptoms including fatigue, balance problems, muscle weakness, and difficulty with coordination and speech. It is a condition that can be incredibly debilitating, and one that can make it difficult for people to live their lives to the fullest.

For many people with MS, the diagnosis can come as a shock. They may have been experiencing symptoms for some time, but they may have been unaware of the severity of their condition. Once diagnosed, they may feel a sense of fear and uncertainty about what the future holds. They may worry about how they will manage their symptoms, and how their condition will impact their relationships, their work, and their daily life.

However, the book "Overcoming Multiple Sclerosis" offers a ray of hope for those living with this condition. Written by someone who has lived with MS for many years, the book provides practical advice and guidance for managing the symptoms of the condition and living a full and active life. The author shares their personal experience with MS, providing insights and strategies that can help others to navigate the challenges of the condition.

The book is designed to be a comprehensive resource for anyone living with MS. It covers a wide range of topics, from diet and exercise to medication and alternative therapies. It emphasizes the importance of taking a holistic approach to managing the condition, focusing not just on the physical symptoms but also on the emotional and psychological aspects of living with a chronic illness.

One of the key messages of the book is that people with MS have a great deal of control over their condition. By making lifestyle changes and adopting healthy habits, it is possible to manage the symptoms of the condition and to live a full and active life. The book offers a wealth of practical advice for making these changes, from tips on healthy eating to suggestions for exercise routines that are safe and effective for people with MS.

Perhaps one of the most valuable aspects of the book is its focus on empowerment. It encourages readers to take an active role in managing their condition, to be informed and engaged in their healthcare, and to advocate for themselves. By taking control of their condition in this way, readers can gain a sense of agency and control, and can feel more confident and capable in the face of the challenges posed by MS.

CHAPTER ONE

Understanding Multiple Sclerosis

The central nervous system, which includes the brain and spinal cord, is affected by the chronic autoimmune disease known as multiple sclerosis (MS).

It is a condition in which the immune system wrongly targets the myelin, the protective layer that surrounds nerve fibers, causing harm to numerous areas of the nervous system. When the myelin is damaged, the transmission of nerve impulses throughout the body is compromised, which interferes with the brain's ability to communicate with the rest of the body.

Since MS is a progressive condition, the myelin loss can worsen with time and result in a wide range of symptoms. Each person will experience MS symptoms differently, but they can include fatigue, tingling or numbness, muscle weakness, balance and coordination issues, vision issues, cognitive impairment, and emotional changes.

The disease's course varies greatly from person to person, with some experiencing just minor symptoms that have little affect on their everyday lives and others possibly dealing with severe, incapacitating symptoms. Relapsing-remitting MS can also have phases in which the symptoms can temporarily get better or even go away, followed by relapses in which the symptoms get worse.

Females are affected by MS at a higher rate than males, and it is most frequently diagnosed in young adults between the ages of 20 and 40. MS is thought to be brought on by a combination of genetic and environmental factors, while its specific cause is still unknown.

Overall, MS is a complicated, frequently unpredictable illness that can have a major influence on a person's life. Although there is no known cure for MS, there are numerous therapies and treatments that can help control symptoms and enhance quality of life for those who have the condition.

Causes of MS

There is still much to learn about the precise causes of multiple sclerosis (MS). Yet, scientists have identified several variables that may play a role in the disease's onset, such as genetics, environmental factors, and immune system abnormalities.

Genetics

Research have revealed that those who come from families where MS has a history are more likely to get the condition. Even though no one gene specifically causes MS, scientists think that some genes may increase a person's risk of getting the condition. In actuality, fraternal twins or non-identical siblings have a lower risk of contracting MS than do identical twins of a person with MS.

Environmental Factors

Environmental elements like bacteria, viruses, and poisons have also been connected to the emergence of MS. For instance, according to some experts, the immune system may be triggered to target the myelin sheath that protects nerve fibers in the central nervous system after being exposed to specific viruses, such as the Epstein-Barr virus.

The chance of having MS may also be increased by other environmental factors such smoking, vitamin D insufficiency, and exposure to solvents or heavy metals.

Immune System Abnormalities

MS is considered to be an autoimmune illness, which means that the body's tissues are wrongly attacked by the immune system. The myelin sheath, which is crucial for the healthy operation of the neurological system, is attacked by the immune system in MS. The immune system attacking the myelin sheath is thought to be caused by immune system anomalies, such as an inefficient T-cell response or an overproduction of certain immune cells.

Moreover, several risk factors have been linked to a higher likelihood of having MS, including:

Age: People between the ages of 20 and 40 are the most frequently diagnosed with MS.

Gender: MS is more likely to affect women than men.

Ethnicity: Those of Northern European ancestry tend to have MS more frequently than those of Black or Asian ancestry.

Geography: MS is more prevalent in regions that are farther from the equator and less prevalent in regions that are nearer the equator.

Although the exact origins of MS are not yet known, ongoing research is shedding light on the intricate interactions between genetics, environment, and the immune system that may play a role in the disease's development. Researchers seek to find a solution for MS, a chronic and frequently crippling disease, by better understanding the underlying causes of the condition.

Types of MS

There are various varieties of multiple sclerosis (MS), and each one has unique traits and patterns of disease development. These kinds of MS can be roughly divided into four basic subtypes: Relapsing-Remitting MS, Primary-Progressive MS, Secondary-Progressive MS, and Progressive-Relapsing MS.

Relapsing-Remitting MS

Around 85% of those with MS have relapsing-remitting MS (RRMS), which is the most prevalent form of the illness. Individuals with RRMS undergo MS relapses, or flare-ups, followed by intervals of remission, during which the symptoms get better or go away. Other classifications for RRMS include active or dormant, as well as with or without signs of illness development.

Primary-Progressive MS

About 10% of MS patients have primary-progressive MS (PPMS), a less prevalent subtype of the illness. In contrast to RRMS, PPMS patients report a steady progression of MS symptoms over time without any relapses or remissions. PPMS can also be divided into two additional categories: active and not active, as well as showing or not showing signs of illness development.

Secondary-Progressive MS

Those who previously had RRMS frequently acquire secondary-progressive MS (SPMS), a form of MS. With SPMS, the disease advances steadily over time, with or without relapses, and symptoms frequently gradually get worse. Relapses may still occur in people with SPMS, but they do so less frequently and with decreasing severity over time.

Progressive-Relapsing MS

Less than 5% of MS patients have progressive-relapsing MS (PRMS), the least common subtype of the illness. In PRMS, the illness proceeds slowly from the start, although the patient also occasionally experiences relapses of symptoms. These relapses could sometimes be followed by fresh symptoms that don't completely go away when in remission.

Due to each type's distinct symptomatology and pattern of disease progression, the various kinds of MS might pose significant problems for those who have the condition. To create a suitable treatment plan, assist MS patients in managing their symptoms, and enhance their quality of life, healthcare providers must make an accurate diagnosis of the kind of MS.

Ultimately, even though each variety of MS has unique traits, it is vital to keep in mind that MS is a complicated and frequently unpredictable disease. Working together with medical specialists to create a tailored treatment plan that takes into account each person's particular requirements and goals is essential because every person with MS experiences the disease differently.

Symptoms of MS

Muscle weakness, balance issues, vision issues, exhaustion, cognitive decline, and sensory abnormalities are just a few of the symptoms of MS, which can vary greatly depending on where and how severely the nerve system has been damaged. Other symptoms include fatigue and eye problems. These signs and symptoms, which can be moderate to severe, can significantly affect a person's daily life and capacity for doing daily duties.

Muscle Weakness and Stiffness

MS frequently manifests as muscle stiffness and weakness. Moving about may be challenging, and speech and other motor functions may also be impacted. In addition to muscle weakness, many MS patients also endure unpleasant and bothersome muscle spasms and tremors. Any area of the body can experience these symptoms, but the arms and legs frequently show them off the most.

Difficulty with Coordination and Balance

Balance and coordination issues are another typical MS symptom. This may make it difficult to walk and raise the possibility of falling. Some MS patients also have a loss of sensation in their limbs, which can make it challenging for them to perceive where their body is with other objects and can further exacerbate balance and coordination issues.

Vision Problems

Blurred or double vision, eye pain, and even momentary vision loss are all common MS symptoms related to vision. Damage to the optic nerve, a typical location of inflammation in MS, may be the source of these symptoms. Moreover, some MS patients may struggle to regulate their eye movements or have uncontrollable eye movements.

Fatigue

Another typical MS symptom is fatigue, which can be both physical and mental. Even after a restful night of sleep, many MS sufferers report feeling weary. As a result of this exhaustion, they may find it challenging to complete daily duties. The most crippling MS symptom in some circumstances, fatigue can have a big influence on someone's quality of life.

Cognitive Impairment

Cognitive impairment, which includes issues with memory, attention, and decision-making, is another prevalent symptom of MS. Some MS sufferers struggle to speak effectively and may have trouble choosing the right words to convey themselves. Cognitive impairment can vary in severity, sometimes being moderate and not having much of an influence on a person's everyday life, other times being more severe and affecting a person's ability to work or carry out other responsibilities.

Sensory Changes

Another typical MS symptom is sensory alterations, which can include numbness or tingling in the face, limbs, or other areas of the body. Burning in the limbs is another symptom experienced by some MS patients, which can be upsetting and inconvenient. These sensory changes can interfere significantly with a person's everyday life and may be sporadic or constant.

Bladder and Bowel Problems

Urinary incontinence, urgency, and trouble emptying the bladder are just a few of the bladder and bowel issues that can occur in MS patients. Moreover, some MS patients may struggle to manage their bowel movements or develop constipation. These symptoms can be embarrassing and have a big effect on how well someone is living.

The signs and symptoms of MS can differ greatly from person to person and fluctuate over time. While some MS sufferers may go through cycles of remission and relapse during which their symptoms come and go, others may endure a more gradual increase of symptoms over time.

Working closely with medical professionals will help MS patients control their symptoms and keep up their general health and wellbeing.

Diagnosis and Management of MS

Given that each person's symptoms differ greatly from one another and frequently resemble those of other neurological conditions, diagnosing and treating multiple sclerosis (MS) can be a complicated and difficult process. Healthcare experts often perform a complete medical history and physical examination, as well as several diagnostic tests, to provide an accurate diagnosis.

Magnetic resonance imaging (MRI), one of the most used MS diagnostic procedures, can assist find the existence of lesions on the brain or spinal cord that are typical with MS. The central nervous system damage's amount and location can be ascertained by medical specialists with the aid of the MRI.

Evoked potential tests, which assess brain electrical activity and can identify irregularities in the transmission of nerve signals, and lumbar punctures, which entail the collection and examination of cerebrospinal fluid, are other procedures that may be used to diagnose MS.

Following an MS diagnosis, medical specialists will collaborate with the patient to create a custom treatment plan that takes into account their unique symptoms and requirements. MS can be treated in a variety of ways, such as with medicine, physical therapy, and lifestyle modifications.

MS symptoms and the disease's course are frequently managed with the aid of medications. In addition to symptom management drugs that can help with specific symptoms like muscle spasms, discomfort, and exhaustion, these medications can also include disease-modifying therapy that aim to lessen inflammation and damage to the myelin sheath in the central nervous system.

Physical therapy can assist to increase mobility, balance, and coordination as well as lessen muscle stiffness and weakness, which can be significant components of controlling MS. Exercises for a particular muscle group's strengthening, balancing exercises, and gait training are all possible components of physical therapy.

Altering one's lifestyle can be a significant part of controlling MS in addition to medical therapy. The severity of MS symptoms may be lessened by eating a healthy, balanced diet, engaging in regular exercise, and minimizing stress. These actions can all assist to enhance general health and wellbeing.

Living with MS can be difficult, but with the appropriate diagnosis and care, many MS sufferers can control their symptoms and lead happy, productive lives. MS patients must collaborate closely with medical providers to create a unique treatment plan that addresses their unique symptoms and needs as well as to make lifestyle adjustments that can enhance their general health and wellbeing. Many MS sufferers can continue pursuing their ambitions and desires and live life to the fullest with the correct care and support.

CHAPTER TWO

The Overcoming Multiple Sclerosis (OMS) Program

To enhance the quality of life for those who have multiple sclerosis, the Overcoming Multiple Sclerosis (OMS) program is a thorough program that promotes lifestyle changes (MS). The program's main goals are to lessen inflammation, encourage neuroprotection, and enhance general health and wellbeing.

It is meant to supplement medical treatment. Doctor and researcher Professor George Jelinek, who was given his MS diagnosis in 1999, is the creator of OMS. Since then, he has made it his mission to share his knowledge and research results with others to assist them in living the best lives they can while dealing with MS.

Science behind the OMS Pprogram

The Overcoming Multiple Sclerosis (OMS) program is supported by a plethora of scientific study and data, notably in the areas of food, exercise, stress management, and supplements. The program's goal is to enhance the health and happiness of MS patients while also perhaps slowing the disease's progression.

Diet

In the OMS program, diet is very important. A plant-based, whole-foods diet with few animal products and saturated fats is advised. This diet is full of whole grains, legumes, fruits, and vegetables, all of which are strong in fiber, antioxidants, and other nutrients that promote overall health and reduce inflammation.

The OMS program also advises staying away from dairy, red meat, and processed foods because these have been known to worsen MS symptoms by causing more inflammation.

Supplements

The OMS program makes extensive use of supplements to promote general health and wellbeing. Because vitamin D, vitamin B12, and omega-3 fatty acids have been found to have neuroprotective effects and reduce inflammation, the program advises taking these supplements.

Exercise

Exercise has been found to improve MS symptoms and is a crucial part of the OMS program. Regular moderate-intensity exercise, such as walking, swimming, or yoga, is encouraged by the program. Exercise helps lessen fatigue and depression while also enhancing strength, balance, and coordination.

Stress Management

An essential element of the OMS program is stress management. Stress can worsen MS symptoms and harm general health and wellbeing. To relieve tension and encourage relaxation, the program suggests employing strategies including mindfulness training, breathing exercises, and meditation.

Sunlight Exposure

Another crucial element of the OMS program is exposure to sunlight. Vitamin D, which is crucial for overall health and has been demonstrated to have neuroprotective benefits, is mostly obtained through sunlight. The program advises spending time outside each day and, if necessary, taking a vitamin D pill.

The OMS program is made to be adaptable so that it may be customized to meet the needs and interests of each individual. Additionally, the program is evidence-based and backed by studies that demonstrate its efficacy in lowering MS symptoms and enhancing general health and wellbeing.

The OMS program's emphasis on fostering long-term health and well-being rather than just controlling symptoms is one of its distinctive features. The program encourages people to actively participate in their care and stresses the value of approaching health and wellness holistically.

In addition, the OMS program is intended to supplement medical care. The program advises against discontinuing or altering any medical therapy without first seeking advice from a healthcare provider. To improve general health and wellbeing, the OMS program can be utilized in conjunction with medical care.

Generally speaking, the OMS program is a thorough lifestyle modification program created to enhance general health and wellbeing in MS patients. The curriculum is supported by scientific research and stresses the significance of approaching health and wellness holistically.

The course is adaptable and may be customized to meet individual requirements and interests. The OMS program provides a distinctive and efficient method for controlling MS symptoms and enhancing quality of life by putting a focus on lowering inflammation, encouraging neuroprotection, and supporting general health and wellbeing.

Benefits of following the OMS Program

For those with multiple sclerosis, following the Overcoming Multiple Sclerosis (OMS) program provides many advantages (MS). Listed below are a few of the primary advantages:

Slowing disease progression

The OMS approach places a strong emphasis on the value of lowering bodily inflammation, which is a major contributor to MS progression. The program can aid in slowing the progression of MS by encouraging regular exercise and stress-reduction measures, as well as eating a diet rich in whole, plant-based foods and low in processed foods and saturated fats.

Reduced relapse rate

The frequency and severity of MS relapses can both be decreased by adhering to the OMS regimen. The program can aid in preventing relapses and lessening their effects when they do happen by lowering inflammation and fostering general health and well-being.

Improved mobility and physical function

Although MS can affect physical function and mobility, a crucial part of the OMS program is frequent exercise. Strength, balance, and coordination can all be enhanced by this, which will enhance physical function and mobility.

Better bladder and bowel function

While MS can also affect bowel and bladder functioning, the OMS program includes strategies like pelvic floor exercises and hydration management to aid with these issues.

Improved energy levels

By encouraging better sleep, lowering stress, and giving the body the nutrients it needs to perform at its peak, the OMS program can help increase energy levels.

Better mental clarity

The OMS program incorporates strategies like mindfulness meditation to help with improving mental focus and clarity, even if MS can also influence cognitive function.

Improved mental health

A person's mental health may suffer as a result of the difficulties and stress that come with living with MS. Following the OMS program, which incorporates stress-reduction exercises like yoga and meditation, can enhance mental health and lessen depressive and phobic symptoms.

Improved social well-being

The OMS program uses strategies like social support groups to assist people with MS connect with others who are going through similar situations, however MS can also influence social well-being.

Following the OMS program can result in an overall increase in the quality of life for people with MS, in addition to these advantages for physical and mental health. The program tackles all facets of health and well-being and gives participants the tools they need to live their best lives with MS by putting a strong emphasis on a complete lifestyle approach.

CHAPTER THREE

Diet and Nutrition

Food and nutrition are crucial elements of wellbeing and good health. A nutritious, well-balanced diet gives the body the nutrition it needs to function correctly and can help stave against several chronic illnesses. In the case of MS, a nutritious diet can be very helpful in controlling symptoms and raising quality of life.

According to studies, some dietary components may increase the likelihood of getting MS, as well as the severity and course of the condition. For instance, research has indicated that a diet high in red meat, dairy products, and saturated fats may raise the chance of developing multiple sclerosis (MS), whereas a diet high in fruits, vegetables, and omega-3 fatty acids may act as a protective factor.

Several research have looked into how nutrition affects MS symptoms and disease progression in addition to how it affects MS risk. According to one study, MS patients' quality of life and fatigue were both reduced when they followed a low-fat, plant-based diet. A diet rich in omega-3 fatty acids, according to another study, was linked to a slower rate of illness development.

Despite mounting data, there is still much that is not known about how diet and nutrition relate to MS. For instance, it is unclear how exactly nutrition affects MS risk and progression or which particular dietary elements are particularly crucial. Also, more study is required to discover the best dietary strategy for MS patients.

Overall, the data point to a possible critical role for a healthy, balanced diet in treating MS symptoms and raising quality of life. But, it's crucial to collaborate with a registered dietitian or healthcare provider to create a customized nutrition strategy that takes into account dietary needs and preferences.

Explanation of the OMS Diet Principles

The OMS diet emphasizes the use of foods that are thought to be good for people with MS and is a whole-foods, plant-based diet low in saturated fat. Dr. George Jelinek, an Australian researcher and physician who was given the MS diagnosis in 1999, created the OMS program.

Based on his own experience with MS and research on the connection between nutrition and MS, Dr. Jelinek created the OMS program. The OMS diet adheres to several fundamental concepts that are intended to assist MS sufferers in controlling their symptoms and enhancing their general well-being. The OMS diet's guiding ideas are as follows:

Elimination of dairy products

Dairy products are prohibited from the OMS diet because they are thought to be a source of saturated fat and a possible MS symptom trigger. A high consumption of saturated fat has been linked to an increased risk of MS, and some MS patients claim that dairy products make their symptoms worse.

Low-saturated fat intake

The OMS diet contains less saturated fat, which is present in meat, dairy, and eggs and other animal products. The diet, on the other hand, places a strong emphasis on the consumption of plant-based foods that are low in saturated fat, like fruits, vegetables, whole grains, legumes, and nuts. Healthy fats like avocado and olive oil are also encouraged by the OMS diet.

Increased consumption of omega-3 fatty acids

Foods high in omega-3 fatty acids, such as flaxseed, chia seeds, walnuts, and fatty fish like salmon and mackerel, are encouraged as part of the OMS diet. It is thought that omega-3 fatty acids contain anti-inflammatory characteristics, which may assist to lessen MS-related inflammation.

Vitamin D supplementation

As vitamin D insufficiency has been associated with an increased risk of MS, the OMS diet suggests regular vitamin D supplementation. Research has indicated that vitamin D may have a preventive impact against multiple sclerosis and is necessary for keeping strong bones and muscles.

Limitation of processed foods and sugar

Processed foods and sugar are restricted on the OMS diet since it is thought that they promote inflammation and may be detrimental to general health. Consuming unprocessed, entire foods including fruits, vegetables, whole grains, legumes, and nuts is encouraged by the OMS diet.

Exercise

The OMS program places a strong emphasis on the value of consistent exercise in treating MS symptoms and enhancing general health, while this is not exactly a dietary principle. People with MS have been proven to benefit from exercise in a variety of ways, including increases in strength, balance, and fatigue.

Several MS patients have experienced improvements in their symptoms and quality of life by following the OMS diet, despite the paucity of evidence on the diet's efficacy. A low-fat, plant-based diet may help with MS symptoms, according to some studies, although additional analysis is required to substantiate these claims.

The OMS diet may not be suitable for all MS patients, so it's crucial to engage with a healthcare provider or certified dietitian to create a customized nutrition plan. The OMS program also incorporates additional lifestyle components, like as stress reduction and mindfulness, that are intended to enhance the general health and wellness of MS patients.

Many MS patients have been able to control their symptoms and enhance their general quality of life by adhering to the OMS regimen.

Importance of Diet in Managing MS

Although there is no known treatment for MS, there are some options that can help control symptoms and halt the disease's development. Maintaining a nutritious diet is vital for managing MS.

According to research, there is a direct correlation between food and MS. While some dietary components may aid in the management of symptoms and enhancement of general health, others may contribute to the onset and development of MS. Some of the most significant ways that diet can help with MS management include the ones listed below:

Managing inflammation

A major contributing element to the onset and development of MS is inflammation. Some diets, such as those rich in sugar and saturated fat, might exacerbate MS symptoms by causing inflammation. A diet high in anti-inflammatory foods, such as fruits, vegetables, whole grains, and omega-3 fatty acids, on the other hand, can aid in reducing inflammation and enhancing general health.

Supporting immune function

Because MS is an autoimmune condition, the body's immune system targets healthy tissue. A balanced diet can lower the likelihood of autoimmune activity and support immunological function. Fruits, vegetables, and whole grains are examples of foods abundant in vitamins and minerals that can strengthen the immune system and lower the risk of problems from MS.

Managing weight

For those who have MS, maintaining a healthy weight is crucial because being overweight can exacerbate symptoms and raise the risk of complications. A nutritious diet reduced in sugar and saturated fat can aid in weight control and enhance general health.

Supporting bone health

Osteoporosis and other bone-related diseases are more common in people with MS. Dairy products and leafy greens are examples of foods high in calcium and vitamin D that can improve bone health and lower the risk of problems.

Managing bowel function

Many bowel-related symptoms, including constipation and diarrhea, can be brought on by MS. The risk of problems can be decreased and bowel function can be managed with a balanced diet rich in fiber.

Tips for Implementing the OMS Diet

If you are interested in implementing the OMS diet, the following tips can help you get started:

Educate yourself

It's critical to educate yourself on diet principles and how to apply them in your daily life before beginning any new dietary regimen. On the organization's website, you may find a variety of information regarding the OMS diet, as well as guides to meal planning, grocery shopping, and cooking.

Eliminate dairy products

Milk, cheese, and yogurt are among the dairy products that must be avoided when following the OMS diet. Dairy products are a major element in many diets, therefore for some people, this can be difficult. Fortunately, there are lots of dairy-free options available, including milks, cheeses, and yogurt made from plants.

Increase consumption of fruits and vegetables

Fruits and vegetables are emphasized as part of the OMS diet because they are full of vitamins, minerals, and antioxidants that can support general health. To ensure that you are getting a variety of nutrients, try to eat at least five servings of fruits and vegetables every day. To do this, choose a variety of various varieties and colors.

Choose healthy fats

The OMS diet places a strong emphasis on consuming good fats, like those in nuts, seeds, avocados, and oily seafood like salmon. These fats can aid in lowering body inflammation and are crucial for maintaining good brain health.

Plan ahead

Following the OMS diet can benefit from meal planning and preparation. To make sure you have everything you need on hand, set aside time each week to plan your meals and snacks. You should also develop a grocery list. To save time over the week, think about batch cooking your meals and snacks.

Seek support

It can be difficult to modify one's diet, therefore talking to people who have similar eating habits might be supportive. If you want to exchange ideas, recipes, and suggestions with others, think about joining an OMS support group or connecting online.

Using the OMS diet is only one part of controlling MS; it's crucial to collaborate with your doctor to create an all-encompassing treatment strategy that takes into account all aspects of your health. While dietary changes can be helpful for many MS sufferers, they should be combined with other therapies and way of life adjustments including stress reduction and consistent exercise.

Meal Planning and Preparation

Using the OMS diet requires careful meal planning and preparation. Here are some pointers for effective meal preparation and planning:

Plan your meals

Plan your meals for the following week each week by blocking off some time. Consider your schedule while you prepare meals, and include quick-to-make options for days when you're busy. To keep your meals interesting and diverse, think about experimenting with different dishes.

Make a grocery list

Make a grocery list of all the things you'll need once you've planned your meals. When you go shopping, stick to your list to prevent making impulsive purchases of processed or unhealthy foods.

Batch-cook meals and snacks

You may save time during the week and make sure you always have wholesome meals and snacks on hand by batch cooking your meals and snacks. To make quick lunches or dinners, think about preparing a big batch of soup or chili. For convenient snacking, you can also pre-cut veggies or prepare a large quantity of hummus or other dips.

Prep ingredients in advance

If batch cooking meals isn't an option for you, think about preparing the components beforehand. Vegetables can be pre-chopped and kept in the refrigerator for quick stir-fries or salads, for instance. For quick meal preparation, you may also pre-cook grains like quinoa or brown rice and keep them in the refrigerator or freezer.

Invest in good storage containers

Planning and preparing meals can be facilitated by using high-quality storage containers. Look for containers with distinct compartments for various foods that are freezer and microwave safe. Glass containers are a wonderful choice because they can be heated in the oven or microwave and are reusable.

Freeze leftovers

If you have any leftover food from a meal, you might want to freeze it for later use. When you don't have time to cook because of your busy schedule, this can be extremely useful. Reheat the leftovers in the microwave or oven after letting them thaw overnight in the refrigerator.

You can make it simpler to follow the OMS diet and make sure you are obtaining the nutrients you need to support your health by taking the time to plan and prepare your meals.

CHAPTER FOUR

Exercise and Movement

The central nervous system is affected by multiple sclerosis (MS), a long-term neurological condition. Muscle weakness, spasticity, issues with balance and coordination, weariness, and soreness are just a few of the symptoms it might produce. To increase strength, flexibility, balance, and general quality of life for those with MS, exercise and mobility have been demonstrated to be useful.

However, depending on the individual's specific symptoms and level of disability, the type and intensity of exercise that is suitable for people with MS may vary. This chapter will address some of the recommended exercise kinds that can be useful in controlling MS symptoms as well as the advantages of exercise and movement for people with MS.

We will also go over some of the difficulties that people with MS could have when trying to exercise and offer advice for overcoming these difficulties.

Role of Exercise in Managing MS

For MS sufferers, regular exercise has a variety of advantages. These are a few ways that exercise can aid in the treatment of the disease's symptoms:

Improve physical function

MS can impair a person's ability to move and carry out daily tasks by causing muscle weakness, stiffness, and decreased coordination. Strength, flexibility, and balance can all be improved with regular exercise, which helps improve physical function and lower the risk of falling.

Workout regimens that emphasize stretching, balance drills, and strength training can be very beneficial for MS patients. While balance exercises can enhance coordination and lower the chance of falling, strength training exercises can assist develop and maintain muscle strength. Stretching activities can assist improve flexibility and alleviate muscle stiffness.

Reduce fatigue

A common MS symptom that can have an impact on a person's quality of life is fatigue. Exercise has been demonstrated to help patients with MS feel less worn out and more energized.

Exercise has been demonstrated to boost the body's utilization of oxygen, which can assist lessen weariness. Those with MS may find that aerobic exercise, such as cycling or walking, is very useful at reducing fatigue. Workout regimens that combine both strength training and aerobic activity may be very useful.

Improve mood

MS can have an impact on a person's emotional health as well, resulting in symptoms like anxiety and despair. In MS patients, exercise has been demonstrated to elevate mood and lessen anxiety and depressive symptoms.

Exercise can help raise levels of endorphins and other neurotransmitters linked to a pleasant mood, according to research. Exercise can also provide MS sufferers a sense of accomplishment and make them feel like they have greater control over their lives.

Slow disease progression

Exercise can help delay the progression of MS by lowering inflammation and supporting neuroprotective mechanisms in the brain and nervous system, even if it cannot treat MS.

Exercise has been linked to a reduction in bodily inflammation, which is thought to contribute to MS onset and progression, according to research. Growth factors that aid in the protection and repair of CNS nerve fibers may also be produced as a result of exercise.

Improve overall health

Frequent exercise can also help to enhance general well-being, lower the chance of developing other illnesses like diabetes and heart disease, and improve overall health.

Many health advantages of exercise have been established, including enhanced mental and cardiovascular health, decreased risk of chronic diseases, and enhanced cardiovascular health. Exercise can help MS sufferers live healthier, more fulfilling lives.

Exercise should be adapted to each person's capabilities and limitations, it is crucial to remember. Before beginning any exercise program, people with MS should speak with a healthcare provider, such as a physical therapist or a certified exercise specialist with experience in MS. A healthcare professional can assist in creating a suitable fitness program that fits the person's needs and goals, as well as monitor progress and make necessary program adjustments.

Exercises Recommended for People with MS

Several forms of exercise are advised for MS patients, depending on their particular symptoms, level of physical fitness, and general health. Some of the most popular workout recommendations for MS sufferers are listed below:

Aerobic exercise

Any form of exercise that raises your heart rate and quickens your breathing is referred to as aerobic exercise or cardio exercise. Walking, cycling, swimming, dancing, and utilizing an elliptical machine are a few examples of aerobic exercise. Those with MS can benefit from aerobic exercise by having more energy, a better cardiovascular system, and less fatigue. Regular aerobic exercise has been found to enhance cognitive performance, mood, and general quality of life in MS patients.

Strength training

To challenge your muscles and increase muscle strength, strength training exercises use resistance, such as weights or resistance bands. Strength training can aid MS patients' physical function and lower their chance of falling. Squats, lunges, bicep curls, and tricep extensions are a few examples of strength training activities. Those with MS who have weakness in their arm or leg muscles may find that strength training is very beneficial.

Balance exercises

Balance training can assist persons with MS gain better coordination and lower their risk of falling. Walking heel to toe, standing on one leg, Tai Chi, and yoga are all examples of balance exercises.

Exercises that improve balance can be especially beneficial for MS patients who have mobility or gait issues.

Stretching exercises

People with MS can benefit from stretching exercises by becoming more flexible and reducing muscle stiffness. Both static stretches, such hamstring or shoulder stretches, and dynamic stretches, like walking lunges or leg swings, can be used as stretching exercises. Exercises that stretch the muscles can be especially beneficial for MS patients who have stiffness or tightness in their muscles.

Pilates

Pilates is a low-impact workout method that emphasizes strengthening the core muscles, developing flexibility, and improving posture. For MS patients who have weakness in their back or abdominal muscles, Pilates can be especially beneficial. Moreover, Pilates helps enhance coordination and balance.

Water exercise

Those with MS who struggle with weight-bearing exercise because of muscular weakness or joint pain may find that water exercises like swimming or water aerobics are an excellent alternative. While still offering cardiovascular and strength-building advantages, water exercise can offer a low-impact workout that is easy on the joints.

It is crucial to remember that the kind and level of exercise should depend on the capabilities and restrictions of each person. Before beginning any exercise program, people with MS should speak with a healthcare provider, such as a physical therapist or a certified exercise specialist with experience in MS. A healthcare professional can assist in creating a suitable fitness program that fits the person's needs and goals, as well as monitor progress and make necessary program adjustments.

Exercise has numerous physical and psychological advantages for MS patients in addition to the physical advantages. Exercise regularly has been demonstrated to elevate mood, lessen stress and anxiety, and enhance general quality of life. Exercise can also boost confidence and self-esteem, which is beneficial for MS patients who might feel constrained by their illness.

Overall, changing one's lifestyle to include exercise can be quite beneficial for those with MS. It can enhance bodily performance and assist with symptom management.

Developing an Exercise Routine

The management of multiple sclerosis (MS) symptoms can benefit from establishing an exercise regimen. Yet, it's crucial to approach exercise with caution and attention. You should also collaborate with a healthcare practitioner to design an exercise program that is both safe and beneficial for you. The following actions can be taken to establish an exercise program for people with MS:

Consult with a healthcare professional

It's crucial to speak with a healthcare expert, such as a physical therapist or a certified exercise specialist with knowledge in MS, before beginning any exercise program. They may assist you in determining your fitness objectives, determining your present fitness level, and creating an exercise regimen that is suitable and safe for you.

Set realistic goals

Setting realistic goals that take into account your present level of fitness and any potential MS-related restrictions is crucial. This can entail beginning with low-intensity activities and progressively boosting the intensity and length over time.

Choose exercises that are safe and appropriate

It's crucial to take your MS symptoms and any physical restrictions into account while selecting workouts. For instance, if you have balance problems, you might want to concentrate on balancing activities like Tai Chi or yoga. Start with low-intensity workouts, such as walking or swimming, if you feel fatigued.

Incorporate a variety of exercises

To increase your general fitness and lower the chance of injury, it's crucial to include a range of activities in your program. This could involve Pilates, stretching, Pilates, balancing drills, and cardiovascular exercise.

Gradually increase intensity and duration

The intensity and duration of your exercises should be gradually increased over time, beginning with a modest level. This will ensure that your training regimen is secure and efficient while also assisting in injury prevention.

Listen to your body

It's crucial to pay attention to your body and modify your training regimen as necessary. It could be important to take a break or alter your exercises if you feel pain or exhaustion. To avoid being too hot, it's also crucial to drink enough of water and take pauses as necessary.

Keep track of your progress

You can keep motivated and on track with your exercise objectives by monitoring your progress. This can be keeping a log of your workouts, using a wearable gadget or fitness app to track your activity, or collaborating with a healthcare expert to track your advancement.

In general, establishing a regular exercise schedule concerning MS can be an important aspect of treating symptoms and enhancing quality of life. You can design a fun and successful fitness program by consulting with a healthcare practitioner, setting reasonable goals, and picking safe and appropriate routines.

CHAPTER FIVE

Stress Management

The management of MS symptoms and enhancement of general wellbeing can both benefit from stress management approaches. This chapter will examine the connection between stress and MS and stress management techniques for MS patients.

We'll talk about several stress-reduction strategies, like mindfulness, relaxation methods, cognitive-behavioral therapy, and exercise, and investigate how they can support people with MS in overcoming the difficulties associated with having this illness. People with MS can enhance their overall quality of life and lessen the negative effects of stress on their physical and mental health by learning effective stress management techniques.

How Stress Impacts MS Symptoms

It is widely known that stress can have a substantial impact on the signs and symptoms of MS. In this post, we'll delve deeper into how stress affects MS symptoms and why stress management is crucial for people with MS.

Stress is a common reaction to a difficult circumstance or incident. It is the body's reaction to a threat or danger that it perceives. Stress causes the body to release hormones like adrenaline and cortisol, which can alter the body's physical and psychological makeup.

While in some circumstances stress can be a normal and healthy reaction, prolonged stress can be harmful to one's physical and mental well-being. Stress can be brought on by many different things for people with MS. The physical signs of the illness can be stressful in and of itself because they might impair independence, movement, and day-to-day activities.

Because MS symptoms can appear and disappear suddenly, its unpredictable nature can also be stressful. However, having a chronic illness can have a tremendous emotional toll and leave one feeling anxious, depressed, and alone.

There are many ways that stress might affect MS symptoms. For instance, stress can contribute to weariness, which is already a typical MS symptom. Stress hormones like cortisol are released by MS patients' bodies when they are under stress, which can affect the immune system and make it harder for the body to fight infections. Increased MS symptoms like weakness, discomfort, and exhaustion may result from this.

Another common MS symptom, spasticity, might be impacted by stress. Involuntary muscular contractions that can result in stiffness, spasms, and pain are what define spasticity. Stress can cause the muscles of people with MS to stiffen up even more, which can worsen the spasticity they already have.

Stress can also affect one's emotions and mental health, which in turn might affect one's MS symptoms. For instance, stress can lead to sadness and anxiety, both of which are typical among MS patients. While depression can result in feelings of melancholy, hopelessness, and apathy, anxiety can lead to feelings of sadness, agitation, and irritation. Anxiety and depression can both have an effect on MS symptoms such fatigue, discomfort, and cognitive impairment.

Effective stress management is crucial for MS sufferers to lessen the negative effects of stress on their physical and mental health. Exercise, mindfulness, relaxation techniques, cognitive-behavioral therapy, and other stress-reduction strategies have all been found to help people with MS cope with stress and live healthier, more fulfilling lives.

Techniques for Managing Stress

A key component of managing multiple sclerosis (MS) is stress management because stress can increase disease symptoms and also cause anxiety, depression, and other psychological problems. Hence, people with MS need to learn a variety of stress management skills and practices that suit them. In this article, we'll go into greater detail about some of the best stress-reduction strategies for MS sufferers.

Mindfulness

Being mindful is a stress-reduction strategy that entails paying attention to one's thoughts, feelings, and physical sensations in the present moment. A potent tool for lowering stress, anxiety, and depression as well as for enhancing general well-being, mindfulness.

There are several ways to exercise mindfulness, including through yoga, meditation, or attentive breathing. The common mindfulness practice of meditation entails finding a peaceful spot to sit, concentrating on the breath, and letting go of any thoughts that may arise. MS sufferers can benefit from meditation's ability to ease stress and encourage relaxation.

Another successful mindfulness method that incorporates both physical activity and attentive breathing and meditation is yoga. Yoga can assist people with MS gain more strength, flexibility, and balance as well as lower their stress levels.

Relaxation techniques

People with MS can reduce stress and improve calm by using relaxation techniques such deep breathing, progressive muscle relaxation, and guided imagery. To help lower pulse rate and soothe the body, deep breathing entails taking long, steady breaths. To help relieve stress and encourage relaxation, different muscle groups are tense and relaxed successively. To relieve stress, guided imagery entails picturing a serene or relaxing picture.

Cognitive-behavioral therapy

Therapy called cognitive-behavioral therapy (CBT) aims to alter unfavorable attitudes and behaviors. For those with MS who are struggling with anxiety or sadness, it can be beneficial. CBT can assist people with MS in recognizing and altering harmful thought patterns that may be causing stress and worry. CBT can help people with MS learn coping mechanisms and stress-reduction practices.

Exercise

For those with MS, exercise is an effective stress-reduction method. Exercise can improve mood, reduce stress, and increase energy levels.. The typical MS symptom of weariness can also be reduced with exercise. People with MS should collaborate with their medical professionals to create an exercise program that is secure and suitable for their requirements and capabilities. Yoga, cycling, swimming, and walking are a few low-impact activities that might be helpful for those with MS.

Social support

By offering emotional support and a sense of belonging, social support can aid people with MS in managing stress. Being a part of a support group or making connections with others who have MS can help lessen feelings of loneliness and give a place to talk about experiences and coping mechanisms. Having social support can also assist MS sufferers keep a positive outlook and enhance their general well-being.

Time management

Stress can be reduced and a sense of control can be fostered with good time management. Prioritizing work, assigning duties, and taking pauses when necessary may be beneficial for MS sufferers. Larger activities can be divided into smaller, more manageable phases to lessen stress and boost productivity.

In conclusion, controlling stress is a key component in managing MS. For people with MS, helpful stress-reduction methods include mindfulness, relaxation techniques, cognitive-behavioral therapy, exercise, social support, and time management. People with MS can enhance their overall quality of life by implementing these tactics into their daily routine and reducing the negative effects of stress on their physical and emotional health.

Overall Health Benefits Of Stress Reduction

Reducing stress is essential for general health and wellbeing and can be very beneficial for both physical and mental health. Persistent stress can harm the body and mind and be a factor in several medical disorders and symptoms. Contrarily, stress management strategies can improve stress management, and they may even be able to stop or lessen the consequences of chronic stress. Reducing the likelihood of developing chronic diseases is one of the main advantages of stress reduction.

Heart disease, diabetes, and some types of cancer are just a few of the health concerns that can be exacerbated by long-term stress. This is since stress causes the release of stress hormones like cortisol and adrenaline, which can increase inflammation, raise blood pressure, and disrupt other vital biological functions. People may be able to lower their chance of developing these and other chronic diseases by reducing their stress levels, improving their long-term health results.

Reducing stress not only lowers the risk of chronic diseases but also strengthens the immune system. Those with weakened immune systems are more prone to infections and diseases due to chronic stress. People may be able to boost their immune systems and lower their chance of being sick or infected by doing so. This is crucial for people with disorders like MS, who may already have weakened immune systems and are more susceptible to infections and diseases.

The lowering of stress can benefit mental health as well. Constant stress can make depression and anxiety more severe mental health conditions. People may be able to enhance their mental health and well-being and possibly delay the onset of these diseases by lowering their stress levels. For MS patients who might already be coping with the psychological side affects of the condition, such as anxiety or depression, this is crucial information.

In addition to these health advantages, stress reduction can lengthen and enhance sleep. Persistent stress can make it difficult to fall asleep, which can result in insomnia and other sleep disorders. People may be able to increase the quantity and quality of their sleep by lowering their stress levels, which will likely enhance their general health and well-being. For those who have MS, who frequently experience sleep disruptions, this is very crucial.

Enhancing energy and vitality can also help reduce stress. It can be challenging to participate in daily activities and enjoy life when experiencing chronic stress because it can cause feelings of lethargy and exhaustion. People may be able to boost their energy and vitality by lowering their stress levels, leading to a more active and meaningful existence. For MS patients who may already be suffering with fatigue as a symptom of the condition, this is especially crucial.

Finally, stress reduction can enhance interpersonal interactions. Persistent stress can cause irritation, moodiness, and other bad emotions, which can all contribute to relationship issues. People may be able to enhance their social contacts and have happier interactions with friends, family, and coworkers by lowering their stress levels. This may result in a stronger sense of social connection and support, which in turn may improve general health and wellbeing.

In conclusion, stress management is crucial to good health and wellbeing, especially for people with illnesses like MS. People can have better physical and mental health, greater energy and vitality, and more rewarding interactions with others by lowering their stress levels.

CHAPTER SIX

Sleep and Rest

Rest and sleep are essential for overall health and wellbeing, and they can significantly affect those with multiple sclerosis (MS). MS is a chronic disorder that affects the central nervous system and can cause a variety of symptoms, including as pain, muscular spasms, and bladder problems, which can interfere with rest and sleep.

MS can also make you tired, which can make it challenging to keep a regular sleep schedule and obtain the rest you need to support your general health. This chapter will examine the connection between MS and rest and sleep, as well as the typical sleep problems that MS sufferers have and management techniques for these problems, to improve general health and wellbeing.

Along with strategies for incorporating relaxation into daily living, we will also talk about the significance of relaxation in controlling MS symptoms. People can enhance their general health and quality of life by being aware of how MS affects sleep and rest and taking action to control these problems.

Importance of Getting Enough Sleep for Managing MS

The management of multiple sclerosis (MS), a long-term autoimmune condition that affects the central nervous system, depends on getting enough sleep. MS can result in a variety of physical and psychological symptoms, such as pain, muscular spasms, anxiety, sadness, and issues with the bladder and bowels, that can affect the quantity and quality of sleep. For those with MS, it is especially crucial to prioritize getting adequate restful sleep.

According to research, sleep is crucial to the body's immune system, and sleep deprivation harms immune performance. This is crucial for MS patients because the condition affects the immune system and makes them more vulnerable to infections and other health issues. A lack of sleep can make MS symptoms including fatigue, cognitive decline, and mood swings worse.

Moreover, sleep is necessary for consolidating memories and learning as well as for the repair and restoration of the body's cells and tissues. For people with MS, getting enough sleep can enhance their mood, cognitive performance, and overall quality of life. Additionally, studies point to a potential link between sound sleep practices and both a slowed rate of MS deterioration and relapse risk.

Regrettably, sleep issues plague people with MS frequently; up to 60% of them report sleep disruptions. Insomnia, sleep apnea, restless leg syndrome, and irregular limb movements are all common sleep issues for MS patients. The cycle of poor sleep and decreasing health outcomes can be exacerbated by these sleep disturbances, which can also increase MS symptoms.

Fortunately, there are numerous methods that people with MS can employ to increase the quantity and quality of their sleep. Establishing a regular sleep schedule is one of them, as are creating a relaxing sleeping environment, staying away from stimulating activities before bed, practicing relaxation techniques, and getting medical attention for underlying sleep issues.

People with MS can better manage their symptoms, strengthen their immune systems, and improve their general health and well-being by making sleep a priority and adopting actions to increase the quantity and quality of their sleep.

Tips for Improving Sleep Quality

To effectively manage the symptoms of multiple sclerosis (MS) and to advance general health and wellbeing, one must get adequate restorative sleep. Unfortunately, sleep issues are a common problem for people with MS, and these issues can make their symptoms worse. Here are some suggestions for enhancing sleep in connection to MS:

Establish a regular sleep routine

The body's internal clock is regulated and improved sleep is promoted by going to bed and waking up at the same time each day. It's crucial to keep a regular sleep routine, even on the weekends.

Create a comfortable sleep environment

Improved sleep and relaxation can be encouraged by a cozy sleeping environment. This entails employing cozy bedding, maintaining a cool, dark environment in the space, and reducing noise and other distractions.

Avoid stimulating activities before bedtime

The ability to fall asleep and maintain asleep can be hampered by stimulation before bed. Avoid doing things like watching TV, using electronics, or doing strenuous exercise in the hours before bed.

Engage in relaxation techniques

Deep breathing, progressive muscle relaxation, and meditation are among relaxation techniques that can help you unwind and have a better night's sleep. These methods can be particularly beneficial for MS sufferers who might experience tension or anxiety.

Exercise regularly

For those with MS, exercise can enhance their general health and quality of sleep. However, it's vital to avoid exercising too soon before bed because it can make you more alert and disrupt your sleep.

Avoid caffeine and alcohol

Alcohol and caffeine are known to disrupt sleep. Caffeine-containing beverages like coffee, tea, and soda should be avoided in the hours before night. Although it may aid in falling asleep at first, alcohol can impair sleep later in the night and cause more frequent awakenings.

Discuss medication options with a healthcare provider

Medication may occasionally be required to enhance MS patients' sleep quality. Given that some drugs may mix with other medications or worsen MS symptoms, it is crucial to review medication alternatives with a healthcare professional.

Manage MS symptoms

Sleep disruptions from MS symptoms like pain, stiffness, and bladder issues are possible. To enhance the quality of your sleep, it's critical to successfully control these symptoms using medicine or other treatments.

Consider cognitive behavioral therapy (CBT)

Therapy called cognitive behavioral therapy (CBT) aims to alter unfavorable thought and behavior patterns that may be linked to sleep issues. For people with MS, it can help alleviate insomnia and enhance the quality of their sleep.

Monitor sleep patterns

People with MS can monitor their sleep habits and find things that might be preventing them from getting enough rest by keeping a sleep diary or using a sleep tracking app. Making a successful sleep plan can be aided by the information provided.

How to Prioritize Rest

To effectively manage the symptoms of multiple sclerosis (MS) and to advance general health and wellbeing, one must prioritize relaxation. Fatigue is a common symptom of MS, and it can be made worse by stress and strenuous activity. Hence, it's crucial to create relaxation techniques that can control fatigue and stop MS symptoms from getting worse.

Here are some pointers for emphasizing relaxation and sleep in connection to MS:

Plan for rest periods

It's crucial to schedule breaks throughout the day, particularly when exhaustion is more obvious. This can entail planning a quick nap or just pausing to relax and refuel.

Listen to your body

Pay attention to your body's cues and rest or take breaks as necessary. When exhaustion is more severe, this may entail modifying your activity level or reducing your workload.

Practice mindfulness

Being mindfully present and aware of the present moment is a type of meditation. It can encourage relaxation and lessen stress. Throughout the day, such as during a quick break or while standing in line, mindfulness practices can be used.

Engage in relaxation techniques

Deep breathing, gradual muscle relaxation, and meditation are all examples of relaxation practices that can help people unwind and manage stress. These exercises can be carried out at home or a serene area like a park or a nature trail.

Prioritize self-care

Self-care activities that encourage relaxation and lower stress levels include taking a warm bath, reading a book, or listening to music. It is crucial to give self-care activities a high priority as part of a regular schedule.

Set boundaries

Establishing boundaries about your career, family, and social obligations might help you feel less stressed and encourage relaxation. This can entail declining certain invitations or assigning work to others.

Seek support

Reduce stress and get emotional support by turning to family, friends, or a support group. The importance of this can't be overstated for MS sufferers who might feel depressed or lonely.

People with MS can manage tiredness, lessen stress, and enhance overall quality of life by prioritizing relaxation. It's crucial to create a tailored relaxation plan that includes a range of tactics and pastimes that suit your requirements and preferences.

CHAPTER SEVEN

Medications and Treatments

Although there is currently no cure for MS, there are numerous drugs and treatments that can help control symptoms, halt the progression of the condition, and enhance a person's quality of life. The purpose of MS drugs and therapies is to manage symptoms including fatigue, discomfort, and muscular spasms while also reducing inflammation and protecting nerve fibers.

This chapter will examine the many types of drugs and therapies, such as disease-modifying medicines, symptomatic treatments, and complementary therapies, that are frequently used to treat MS. We will go through each sort of treatment's advantages and disadvantages as well as its administration and monitoring procedures.

We will also discuss the significance of collaborating with a healthcare professional to create a tailored treatment plan that takes into account your particular requirements and preferences. It is crucial to remember that MS drugs and treatments are always changing, and new therapies are always being created and evaluated.

To make sure you are getting the best and most appropriate care, it is essential to stay up to date on the most recent developments in MS therapy and to work closely with your doctor.

Overview of Medications Used to Treat MS

Almost 2.3 million people are thought to have MS worldwide, with women being more afflicted than males. While there is no proven treatment for MS, there are several drugs that can help manage the symptoms and halt the disease's development.

Reducing the number and intensity of MS relapses, delaying the disease's progression, managing symptoms, and enhancing general quality of life are all objectives of MS treatment. It is possible to use a variety of pharmaceutical types to accomplish these objectives.

Interferon beta

For the treatment of relapsing-remitting MS, the drug interferon beta is administered intramuscularly or subcutaneously (RRMS). By inhibiting the immune system, it lessens the frequency and severity of MS relapses. Relapse rates can be decreased by up to 30% with interferon beta, and the disability progression can be slowed. Avonex, Rebif, and Betaseron are a few examples of popular interferon beta brands.

Glatiramer acetate

Treatment for RRMS involves the subcutaneous injection of glatiramer acetate. It functions by preventing the immune system from attacking the myelin that surrounds nerves in the central nervous system and serves as a protective covering. It has been demonstrated that glatiramer acetate can slow the onset of impairment and decrease relapse rates by up to 29%. Glatiramer acetate is marketed under the name Copaxone.

Dimethyl fumarate

Oral dimethyl fumarate is a medicine used to treat RRMS. It functions by lowering inflammation in the central nervous system, which may help the disease advance more slowly. It has been demonstrated that dimethyl fumarate can stop the course of impairment and can cut the number of relapses by up to 50%. Dimethyl fumarate is sold under the trade name Tecfidera.

Fingolimod

Fingolimod is a medicine used to treat RRMS that is administered orally. To lessen the quantity of immune cells that can target the central nervous system, it prevents immune cells from exiting lymph nodes, which is how it functions. It has been demonstrated that fingolimod can slow the onset of impairment and can cut down on relapses by up to 54%. Fingolimod goes under the name Gilenya.

Natalizumab

For the treatment of RRMS, an injectable drug called natalizumab is used. It functions by limiting the number of immune cells that can attack the central nervous system by blocking their passage through the blood-brain barrier. There is evidence that natalizumab can decrease the progression of impairment and cut back on relapses by up to 68%. Tysabri is the brand name for the drug natalizumab.

Alemtuzumab

To treat RRMS, an injectable drug called alemtuzumab is used. It operates by eliminating immune cells that target the brain and spinal cord. According to studies, alemtuzumab can stop the progression of impairment and can cut down on relapses by up to 50%. Alemtuzumab goes by the brand name Lemtrada.

Ocrelizumab

Ocrelizumab is a drug that is given intravenously to treat both primary progressive MS and RRMS (PPMS). It operates by concentrating on immune cells called B cells, which are involved in attacking the central nervous system. Ocrelizumab has been proven to delay the course of disability in both RRMS and PPMS and to cut the number of relapses in RRMS by up to 50%. The first drug for the treatment of PPMS that the FDA has approved is ocrelizumab. A brand name for ocrelizumab is ocrevus.

Mitoxantrone

For the treatment of advanced MS, mitoxantrone is a drug that is given intravenously. By lowering inflammation in the central nervous system and suppressing the immune system, it suppresses infection. However, mitoxantrone has serious possible side effects, such as heart damage and an increased risk of leukemia. It has been demonstrated that mitoxantrone helps to decrease the frequency of relapses and halt the course of impairment.

Corticosteroids

To treat MS relapses, corticosteroids are drugs that can be used orally or intravenously. They function by lessening central nervous system inflammation. Corticosteroids can lessen the frequency and severity of relapses, but they do not influence how quickly the disease develops. Prednisone, methylprednisolone, and dexamethasone are a few typical corticosteroids used to treat MS relapses.

In addition to these medications, various more treatments can be used to manage the symptoms of MS, including medications to reduce spasticity, exhaustion, pain, and bladder dysfunction. Moreover, physical therapy, occupational therapy, and speech therapy can treat speech and swallowing issues as well as mobility, strength, and coordination issues.

The choice of medication for MS therapy will rely on several variables, including the kind and severity of the condition, the patient's medical history, as well as their personal preferences and treatment objectives. Working closely with a healthcare professional is crucial to create a treatment plan that is specific to each patient's requirements and to track the efficiency and side effects of any medications used.

Alternative Therapies and Treatments

Some numerous alternative therapies and treatments can be employed in the management of multiple sclerosis in addition to conventional drugs and therapies (MS).

While some of these treatments might be beneficial for some individuals, it's crucial to remember that they haven't undergone extensive clinical trials to demonstrate their efficacy and may not be suitable for everyone. Patients should consult with their doctor before attempting any alternative therapies or treatments.

Dietary supplements

To control their symptoms or limit the disease's course, some MS patients may use dietary supplements. Omega-3 fatty acids, vitamin D, and antioxidants are examples of supplements that are frequently used. An important aspect of MS is inflammation, which omega-3 fatty acids in fish oil are thought to help with. Low vitamin D levels have been associated with an increased chance of getting MS, hence vitamin D has also been researched concerning the condition.

Antioxidants, such those in berries and green tea, can aid to lower inflammation and enhance general health. Further research is required to assess the usefulness of these supplements in treating MS, even though some studies have suggested that they may be beneficial in lowering inflammation and enhancing general health.

Acupuncture

Thin needles are inserted into certain body spots during the ancient Chinese practice of acupuncture to promote healing and reduce pain. According to certain research, acupuncture may help MS sufferers with their pain, exhaustion, and despair. To ascertain the efficacy of this treatment, more research is required.

Yoga and meditation

Patients with MS may benefit from yoga and meditation because they can lower stress, enhance balance and coordination, and increase flexibility and strength. According to some research, these techniques may also aid with exhaustion, depression, and anxiety. Some MS patients who practice yoga may find their bladder control has improved. It is crucial to remember that some yoga postures, such as those that cause spasticity, may not be suitable for people with certain MS symptoms and should be avoided or adjusted.

Exercise therapy

Patients with MS may benefit from exercise therapy to increase their flexibility, coordination, and muscle strength. Exercise may aid in lowering fatigue and enhancing general quality of life, according to several research. Exercises including resistance training, cardiovascular exercise, and aquatic treatment may be beneficial for MS sufferers. But, it's crucial to collaborate closely with a healthcare professional to create an activity program that is secure and suitable for each patient, as some forms of exercise may make some MS symptoms worse.

Cannabis

It has been suggested that cannabis may be used to alleviate MS symptoms, including pain and spasticity. Cannabis may help manage these symptoms, according to some data, but it is crucial to remember that marijuana also has potential side effects and may interact with other treatments. Patients should be informed of the potential hazards and benefits of cannabis use and should discuss it with their healthcare physician.

Mind-body therapies

Patients with MS may benefit from mind-body therapies like hypnosis, guided imagery, and biofeedback to relieve tension and anxiety. According to some research, these treatments may also aid with pain management and quality of life enhancement. To ascertain whether these treatments are successful for MS, more research is necessary.

Massage therapy

In MS patients, massage therapy may assist to ease tension in the muscles and encourage relaxation. Studies have also suggested that receiving massage treatment may aid with pain management and general quality of life enhancement. However, it is crucial to work with a licensed massage therapist who has experience treating MS patients and to steer clear of massage if there are any particularly sensitive or painful body parts.

Chiropractic care

To enhance general health and reducing pain, chiropractic therapy involves manipulating the spine and other joints. Chiropractic care may help some MS patients with pain management and movement improvement, but it's crucial to work with a skilled chiropractor who has expertise treating MS patients and to avoid any maneuvers that can aggravate MS symptoms.

Cognitive-behavioral therapy

The goal of cognitive-behavioral therapy (CBT), a type of psychotherapy, is to alter unfavorable ideas and behaviors to enhance general mental health. According to several research, CBT may help MS patients with their anxiety, depression, and other psychological problems. The development of coping mechanisms and general quality of life may also benefit from CBT.

Traditional Chinese medicine

Herbs, acupuncture, and other treatments are used in traditional Chinese medicine (TCM) to support general wellness and balance. Although it's crucial to work with a skilled TCM practitioner who has expertise treating MS patients, some MS patients may find TCM useful in lowering symptoms including fatigue, pain, and spasticity. It's also important to avoid any therapies that might combine with other medications.

It is crucial to remember that, even while these complementary therapies and treatments may be beneficial for some individuals, they should never be utilized in place of conventional medical care. To create a thorough treatment plan that includes both conventional and alternative therapies, as well as to track the effects and side effects of any treatments employed, it is imperative to work closely with a healthcare provider.

Also, before starting any new therapy, patients should explore the potential advantages and disadvantages of any alternative medicines with their doctor.

CHAPTER EIGHT

Lifestyle and Social Support

Although there is presently no cure for MS, there are several behavioural modifications and social support strategies that can help patients manage their symptoms, preserve their physical and psychological welfare, and improve their quality of life in general.

This chapter will examine how various lifestyle choices, such as exercise, diet, stress reduction, and quitting smoking, can affect how MS develops. We'll also go through the value of social support in the lives of MS patients and offer tips for creating and sustaining a solid support system.

Patients with MS can enhance their general health and wellbeing by integrating these lifestyle modifications and social support strategies, and they can lead satisfying lives despite the obstacles of their illness.

Strategies for Adapting to Life with MS

MS can make daily life difficult, but with the right care and management, MS sufferers can have happy, fulfilled lives. The following are some tips for adjusting to life with MS:

Obtain routine medical attention

Working closely with your doctor will help you manage your MS symptoms and medication. Your doctor can assist you in developing a treatment strategy that caters to your particular requirements and may include medication, physical therapy, and dietary adjustments.

Manage your symptoms

People with MS can have a wide range of symptoms, but frequent ones include fatigue, numbness, weakness, and issues with balance and coordination. These symptoms can be controlled in a variety of ways, including through exercise, relaxation, stress reduction, and medication.

Stay active

A crucial component of managing MS is exercise. Frequent exercise can help with exhaustion and depression and can also aid with strength, balance, and coordination. See your doctor about creating a personalized workout plan that is both safe and beneficial for you.

Eat a healthy diet

Your entire health and wellbeing can be supported by eating a balanced diet. Consuming a mix of fruits, vegetables, healthy grains, and lean protein sources will assist in giving your body the nutrition it needs to operate at its peak performance.

Manage stress

It's crucial to learn stress management techniques because stress can make MS symptoms worse. This could entail using relaxation methods like meditation or deep breathing, as well as asking friends, family, or a mental health professional for support.

Get support

It's critical to seek out support from others who understand what you're going through because MS may be isolating. This can entail speaking with a therapist, joining a support group, or making internet connections with others.

Plan for the future

Because MS is a progressive disease, making plans is crucial. Making financial arrangements, coming up with a long-term care strategy, or discussing your end-of-life care preferences with close ones are a few examples of what this entails.

It's important to keep in mind that managing MS is a journey with ups and downs. You can adjust to having MS and carry on living a happy life by working closely with your doctor and taking care of yourself.

Importance of Social Support in the Lives of MS Patients

Social support is an important part of managing Multiple Sclerosis (MS). Patients with MS who have a strong support system of family, friends, and medical personnel are better able to handle the difficulties of their condition and enjoy a higher quality of life.

The emotional support that social support offers MS patients is among its most important advantages. Living with a chronic condition like MS can be difficult, and sufferers may feel isolated, lonely, or anxious.

By giving patients a sense of community, acceptance, and understanding, social support can help lessen these emotions. Supportive friends and family members can listen to patients' worries, acknowledge their sentiments, and provide them encouragement and inspiration to keep going.

Another essential component of social support for MS patients is practical support. Help with daily chores like food shopping, meal preparation, and housekeeping might be considered a form of practical support. Practical assistance can significantly improve the quality of life for MS patients who may have physical restrictions or exhaustion.

Also, patients who receive this kind of support may be able to keep their independence and enhance their general quality of life. While the costs of controlling the disease can be high, financial help is especially crucial for MS patients.

Financial strain can make MS-related expenses like medical care, mobility aids, and home renovations even more burdensome. This burden can be lessened and social support in the form of financial assistance, such as assistance with medical costs or assistance finding resources, can help MS patients get the care they require.

MS patients may also gain from engaging in internet forums or support groups where they can interact with others going through comparable circumstances. Support groups can give MS patients a sense of belonging, a forum to express their experiences, and a chance to pick the brains of other patients. Support groups may also provide information about new treatments, clinical trials, and research as educational resources.

In conclusion, MS patients need social support very much. Peer support, financial support, practical aid, and emotional support are all essential in assisting MS sufferers in coping with the difficulties of their condition and enhancing their overall quality of life. To make sure that MS patients have the tools and support they need to properly manage their illness, healthcare practitioners should encourage them to establish and maintain a strong support network.

Building a Support Network

Creating a support system is crucial for MS sufferers. Having a support network in place can ease the trip because MS is a chronic condition that can be difficult to manage. Here are some pointers for creating an MS support system:

Join a support group

A excellent approach to meet people who are going through similar things is through support groups. There are numerous MS support groups available, both offline and online. These groups can offer a secure and encouraging setting where you can express your emotions, ask concerns, and pick up advice from others.

Connect with others online

For those who have MS, there are numerous online forums and communities. These groups can be a valuable source of knowledge, counsel, and assistance. Also, they can provide people a feeling of community and belonging, especially those who might not have access to physical support groups.

Talk to your family and friends

It's crucial to have a reliable support network in your private life as well. Tell your loved ones about your MS and ask them how they can help. This could entail offering emotional support, assisting with everyday duties, or just being there to listen.

Seek professional support

It's vital to seek professional support if necessary because managing MS can be emotionally taxing. To control your emotions and create coping mechanisms, you might do this by speaking with a therapist or counselor.

Educate your loved ones

It's crucial to inform your loved ones about MS and how it affects you because it's a difficult disorder. They will be able to support you in managing your symptoms and better understand your needs as a result of this.

Volunteer or get involved in advocacy

Participating in MS advocacy can be a terrific way to meet new people and change the world. Think about doing volunteer work for an MS organization or taking part in fundraising activities. In addition to assisting others, you'll develop relationships and a sense of purpose.

Keep in mind that creating a support system requires time and effort. It's crucial to be persistent and patient in your attempts to develop connections with other people and form bonds with them. Living with MS may be tolerable and rewarding with the correct support.

CHAPTER NINE

Navigating MS in the Long Term

For many MS patients, controlling the condition necessitates a long-term plan that considers the disease's unpredictable character. Long-term management of MS necessitates a complex strategy that involves consistent medical attention, lifestyle modifications, and a solid support network.

This chapter will discuss how to manage MS over the long term, including the value of routine medical care, symptom management techniques, the impact of food and exercise, and creating a support system. The chapter will also explore the emotional and psychological effects of having MS as well as the value of advocacy and self-care.

Strategies for Planning for the Future

Living with MS can make it difficult to plan for the future because each person is affected by the condition differently and it can be unpredictable. Nonetheless, some methods can assist people with MS in making plans:

Establish financial security

MS may affect a person's capacity to work and generate income, which may affect their financial security. Establishing financial security through savings, disability insurance, and other methods of financial preparation are all examples of future planning.

Make home modifications

MS can affect a person's mobility and capacity for navigating their home. Implementing house modifications can assist people with MS preserve their freedom and safety in their homes by installing grab bars, ramps, and other accessibility features.

Consider career options

MS may affect a person's capacity to work or restrict their job prospects. Investigating job possibilities that are more compatible with a person's strengths and weaknesses can be a part of future planning.

Create a support plan

Making a support plan that specifies who will give care and support if a person's condition worsens can be a part of future planning. To create a plan that is tailored to a person's needs, this may entail collaborating with healthcare professionals, family members, and other support networks.

Consider legal planning

Legal planning, such as drafting a will, power of attorney, and advance directives, may also be a part of future planning. These legal documents can aid in making sure that someone's wishes are carried out and that their affairs are handled properly.

Preparing for the future while living with MS necessitates a thorough strategy that considers a person's medical, emotional, and practical requirements. People with MS can confidently plan for the future and maintain a sense of control over their lives by maintaining regular medical care, creating a support network, establishing financial security, making home modifications, thinking about career options, creating a support plan, and thinking about legal planning.

CONCLUSION

Taking Control of Your Health

A person's quality of life may be significantly impacted by multiple sclerosis (MS), a chronic illness. There is no known cure for MS, however there are numerous things MS patients may do to manage their symptoms and enhance their general health.

Building a relationship with a medical group that specializes in MS care is among the most crucial things MS patients can do. A neurologist, primary care doctor, physical therapist, and additional experts as needed could be a part of this team. A healthcare team can offer direction and support, help MS patients manage their symptoms, and modify their treatment plan as needed.

People with MS can improve their general health through nutrition, exercise, and stress reduction in addition to working with a healthcare team. Consuming a well-balanced diet full of fresh produce, whole grains, and fiber can strengthen the immune system and lessen inflammation.

Frequent exercise can lower the chance of secondary health issues like heart disease and osteoporosis while enhancing mobility, strength, and balance. Meditation, deep breathing, and yoga are all stress-reduction methods that can also enhance general wellbeing.

Acupuncture, massage, and yoga are examples of complementary and alternative therapies that may be beneficial in treating MS symptoms. Although there is little evidence to support these therapy, some MS patients find them helpful in lowering pain, fatigue, and muscular stiffness. Before beginning any complementary or alternative therapy, it's crucial to discuss it with a healthcare practitioner to ensure that it is both secure and efficient.

For those who have MS, it's critical to keep up with the most recent developments in MS research and treatment options. There is a plethora of information on MS and related subjects as well as support and instructional tools available from the National MS Society and other advocacy groups. Sharing knowledge and experiences with others who have MS through internet forums and support groups can also be beneficial.

Finally, a crucial component of treating MS is speaking up for your needs and yourself. This may entail discussing your treatment preferences with your medical team, asking for adjustments at work or in other places, and getting in touch with advocacy groups that can assist you in navigating the difficulties of living with MS.

In summary, controlling MS necessitates a diverse strategy that involves working with a healthcare team, adopting healthy routines, thinking about complementary and alternative therapies, being informed, and speaking up for yourself. Even though MS can be a difficult disease to manage, there are numerous tools and techniques available to support persons with MS in leading meaningful lives. People with MS can enhance their quality of life and preserve their independence for as long as feasible by actively managing their health.

Printed in Great Britain
by Amazon

27430498R00056

ISBN 9798387618840